To everyone that helped me walk again

The Ultimate Guide to Strong Healthy Feet

First Edition

ISBN-13:
978-1518728129

ISBN-10:
151872812X

PRINTED IN THE UNITED STATES OF AMERICA

Medical Disclaimer

The information in this book is not intended or implied to be a substitute for professional medical advice, diagnosis or treatment. All content, including text, graphics, images and information, contained on or available through this book is for general information purposes only. The author makes no representation and assumes no responsibility for the accuracy of the information contained on or available through this book, and such information is subject to change without notice. You are encouraged to confirm any information obtained from or through this book with other sources, and review all information regarding any medical condition or treatment with your physician.

NEVER DISREGARD PROFESSIONAL MEDICAL ADVICE OR DELAY SEEKING MEDICAL TREATMENT BECAUSE OF SOMETHING YOU HAVE READ ON OR ACCESSED THROUGH THIS BOOK.

The author does not recommend, endorse or make any representation about the efficacy, appropriateness or suitability of any specific tests, products, procedures, treatments, services, opinions, health care providers or other information that may be contained on or available through this book.

THE AUTHORS IS NEITHER RESPONSIBLE NOR LIABLE FOR ANY ADVICE, COURSE OF TREATMENT, DIAGNOSIS OR ANY OTHER INFORMATION, SERVICES OR PRODUCTS THAT YOU OBTAIN THROUGH THIS BOOK."

Affiliation and Endorsement Disclaimer

Any product names, logos, brands, and other trademarks or images featured or referred to within this book are the property of their respective trademark holders. These trademark holders are not affiliated with the author, this book, or our website. They do not sponsor or endorse this book or any of our online products. This book declares no affiliation, sponsorship, nor any partnerships with any registered trademarks.

Table of Contents

Morton's Toe **53**

Conclusion **54**

The Problem: Weak Feet

A huge problem that goes nearly unnoticed in society today is that people's feet are extremely weak. Having weak feet can cause a cascade of problems in the foot itself, and elsewhere in the body.

Weak feet cause:

- **Structural issues in the bones/muscles/ligaments of the feet.** Common issues to foot structures are bone fractures (traumatic or repetitive stress induced), faulty bone alignment (bunions), inflammation of tendon or ligament, and muscle tears. When these problems arise, you cannot walk! You feel the pain all day, and it can drive you crazy.

- **Circulation problems in the feet, legs and the rest of the body.** Your body relies on the muscles in your feet and legs to pump blood through them, and back up to the heart (which is tough because it has to pump the blood up the legs, against gravity). If your feet and legs are weak, or not often used (from sitting in chairs all day), then circulation will be hindered. Reduced circulation will result in detrimental effects throughout the body. Also, bad circulation will cause accumulation of waste products around the nerves of the feet, which can cause degeneration and faulty nerve signaling and transmission.

- **Nerve Problems in the feet.** Weak muscles in the feet will cause bones to be out of alignment which can cause nerves to be impinged (pinched). This can cause chronic pain, numbness and burning on the feet.

- **Balance and Coordination Faults.** Your body's sense of balance relies on sensory nerves in the feet to tell the brain where the body is in three-dimensional space. Your feet tell your brain where you are, and this helps the brain control the muscles that allow you to move. If the nerves are not functioning properly, or the muscles are weak, then your balance and coordination will be compromised.

- **Chronic pain and instability in the ankles/knees/hips/back.** The feet are the foundation of many other structures in the body. If the feet are weak, the body will be weak. Everything in the body is connected. Your feet belong to a chain of other structures that rely on each other for strength and functionality. These connected structures are termed "kinetic chains." This is important to understand because when the feet are weak, the bones of the feet/legs/hip/back fall into unfavorable positions.
  When bones are out of alignment, the muscles that attach to the bones will become excessively shortened or lengthened, which will make them weaker (another potential

downward spiral situation: Weak feet cause weak feet). This will also cause various joints to be placed into positions that they were not made to be in, which will make them susceptible to injury. Joints also serve an important purpose in the body for the sensory perception of the body's position. We rely on sensory nerves in the joints to tell the brain what position the joints are in. If the joints are placed in unstable positions for prolonged amounts of time, they will adapt to the position by becoming excessively flexible (lax). This can cause problems with the nerve signals going to the brain, which will later cause problems in muscle control. All of these factors contribute to the development and perpetuation of chronic pain in the ankles/knees/hips and back.

- **Dysfunctional Walking Gait Mechanics.** Having weak feet will always cause unfavorable changes in walking gait (and having bad walking gait will inherently make your feet weaker. This is why foot issues like to become chronic).

- **It is depressing.** Having weak feet is a huge bummer because chronic pain associated with weak feet sucks. Strong feet allow you to stay active and have fun!

These are the main problems, but many more go unnoticed. Many foot problems and associated issues (such as back pain) are unfortunately considered "part of being human." This is how humans justify a problem that they cannot solve. They just give up and say, "that is just the way it is." However, that is not the case! If you feel pain or soreness from basic human activities, something is wrong. You need to fix the cause of the problem and move on with your life.

Why Are They Weak?

Shoes

Shoes are the number one cause of weak feet. Your feet are not made to be in a shoe. Shoes have multiple inherent faults:

1. Shoes elevate the heel of the foot. This is commonly termed "heel elevation".
2. Shoes elevate the toes of the foot upward. This is called "toe spring."
3. Shoes squeeze the toes and bones of the foot together.
4. Shoes compress the blood vessels, lymphatic vessels, and nerves.

These 4 things set forth a cascade of problems in the feet and elsewhere on the body. Let me explain:

1. When shoes force the heel to be elevated, the toes to be bent upwards and squeezed together, you fix the bones into a position that favors pronation (collapsed foot arch). In the picture below, I have raised the heel, the toes, and squeezed the toes together, which has caused the arch to collapse (pronation):

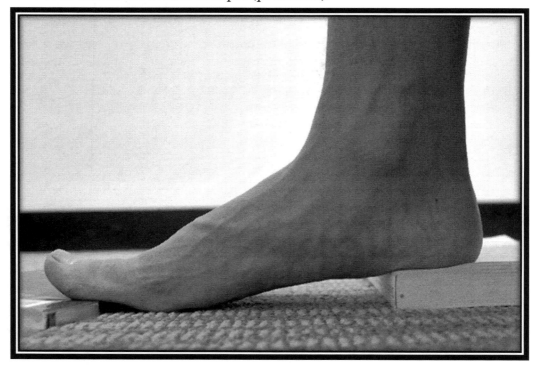

The picture below is a top view of this movement. When the toes get pushed together, and the heel is elevated, the ankle goes inward, and the arch of the foot collapses. This is what happens when you wear shoes.

This is called pronation.

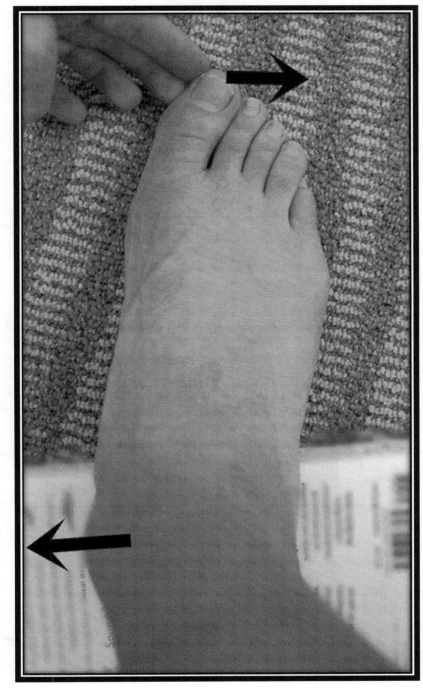

If you take off your shoes, and you plant your heel and toes on the ground and spread out your toes, pronation disappears. The arch rises up, and the muscles of the foot start to engage. This is what your feet are supposed to look like:

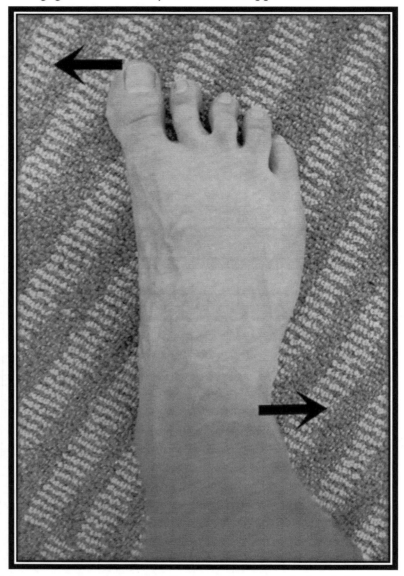

Keep in mind that pronation is good and required to absorb shock from the ground. Pronation is a natural movement required to walk. The problem arises when shoes force the feet into a pronated position all day long. When they are forced into pronation, they cannot absorb shock from the ground. This shock will get distributed to other structures in the body, especially the ankles, knees, hips and back.

2. When the feet are chronically pronated, then the lower leg bones are forced into an excessive internal rotation. This causes the knees to collapse inward, which causes the thigh bone to become internally rotated, which then shifts the pelvis bone into a forward tilt (anterior pelvic tilt). The pelvis is the foundation of your spine. When the pelvis is tilted forward, the spine will be pushed out of alignment (arch in the lower back):

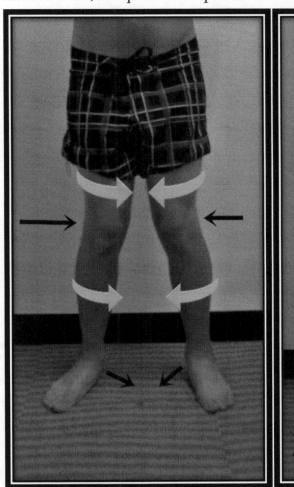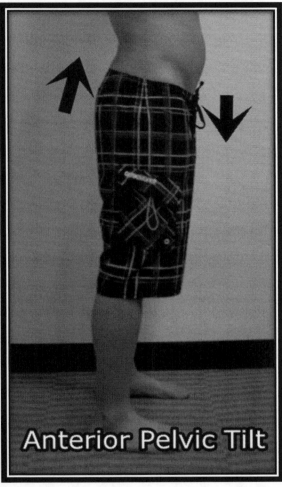

Anterior Pelvic Tilt

When all of these bones are out of alignment, the muscles that attach to them become dysfunctional. Some of them become longer and weak, and some become shorter and inhibited. This is why people have tight calves, tight hamstrings, tight hip flexors and tight back muscles. This is also why their abdominal muscles, glutes, quads and foot extensors are always weak. These muscles are being forced into a dysfunctional position, and the muscles are adapting to it by becoming shorter or longer (weak or inhibited). This is horrible and causes many problems!

3. When the bones and muscles are dysfunctional, then the joints are the next structure to be damaged. For joints to be strong, they need the bones to be in a healthy position, and they need the muscles to be firing correctly and working within their healthy range of motion (not too short, not too long). When the bones and muscles are dysfunctional, it causes your joints to be forced into unstable positions, which is the perfect environment for chronic joint pain to develop. If you have chronic pain in your ankles/knees/hips/back, then pronation caused by shoes is a likely culprit.

The pictures below show what proper pelvic and leg posture is supposed to look like. Notice that the knees are pointed forward and not bending inward. Notice how the arch of the back is less pronounced. Then look at my feet! The arch is raised, and my toes are spaced apart. This is how you humans are made to stand:

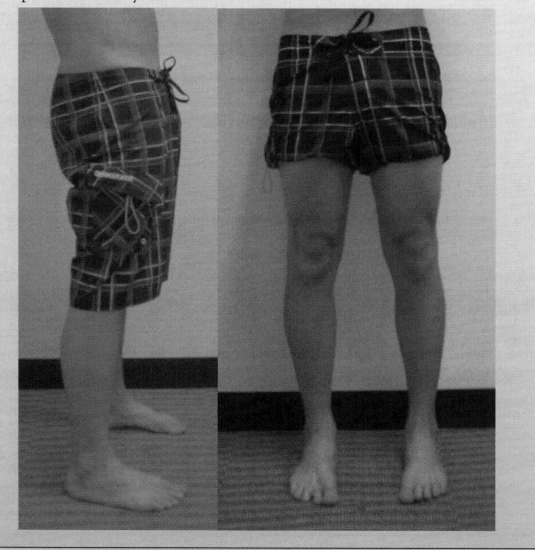

The cascade of problems mentioned a second ago will indirectly lead to further issues:

- Your calf muscles have an elaborate system of valves which cause your blood to be pumped upwards against gravity, so that it can return to your heart, to be pumped elsewhere in the body. When a shoe causes the heel to be elevated, the calf muscles become shortened, which reduces the effectiveness of this system. If you wear a shoe with an elevated heel, circulation for the entire body is reduced.
- Shoes constrict the bones and joints from moving. A healthy and freely mobile foot can absorb the impact from the ground while walking (there are other movements that absorb shock beside pronation). When a shoe holds all the bones in a static and unmovable position, they are unable to absorb shock from the ground, and the force is instead dissipated in the ankles, knees, hips, and back.
- When the bones of your feet are forced into unstable positions, some of your foot muscles become excessively stretched or shortened (as mentioned earlier). Some muscles of the feet are near blood and lymph vessels and nerves. If these muscles are weak or excessively stretched, then they will inhibit the nearby blood/lymph and nerve supply. Reducing blood, lymph and nerve activity can cause problems elsewhere in the feet. Always remember that when an area lacks circulation, then degenerative processes develop, such as Plantar fasciitis, Achilles tendonitis and more.

Understand that athletic shoe companies manipulate people to believe that shoes can be good for their feet. They use features such as motion control, gel cushion, pronation control to make people believe that they are a good choice. Many of the shoes that are promoted as being a "health promoting shoe" actually cause the problems that they were meant to fix. 99% of shoes available today directly cause chronic foot problems. Many people do not realize this because these shoes feel great for the first 3 months that you wear them. These shoes make it possible for the feet to get lazy, and not do their job of stabilizing and supporting the body. Avoid all advice from shoe sales people! If you are one of the few people who has an actual problem that can be corrected with shoes or orthotics, go to a holistic podiatrist or walking gait mechanics professional. Everyone else will waste your time and money.

Too much support

Wearing an arch support such as an orthotic will cause the muscles of the feet to be lazy, which will make them weak. Orthotics also detrimentally reduce impact by distributing force across the entire foot (the foot should only contact the ground at the toes, outside edge of the foot and the heel). Less impact where it is required will cause the bones to weaken. Walking on an arch support can also reduce blood flow to some areas of the feet. They also minimize the ability of the foot to move, which reduces the foot's natural ability to absorb shock.

Many will ask, "Don't I need an arch support to correct pronation?" and the answer is no! Fixing excessive pronation with an arch support will make the problem worse. The best arch support available is strong foot muscles and a properly positioned pelvis.

Sitting in Chairs and Sedentary Lifestyle

Sitting in chairs automatically tilts your pelvis forward. The muscles will then adapt to this position and hold it there. This will cause your thigh bone to rotate internally, your knees to collapse inward, your lower leg bones to internally rotate which causes… Pronation! Sitting in a chair will ultimately cause your feet to pronate excessively, which will cause foot problems.

Sitting in chairs also causes detrimental effects in every organ system of the body. Recent studies have showed that sitting down all day is just as unhealthy as smoking!

If you have a lazy lifestyle that is filled with video games, driving cars and working indoors, there is a good chance that you do not use your feet that much. When you do not use your feet, the bones in your feet become brittle. If you have bone spurs or stress fractures, there is a good chance that your activity levels are to blame (or possibly your diet).

Bad Diet

Your feet are made from the foods you eat. The raw materials and energy that the feet use to survive all come from your diet. If your diet is filled with processed foods or toxic chemicals that cause structural weakness, you are at risk of developing foot problems.

Cold Environment

Having your body maintain its temperature in cold environments is taxing on the body. It will cause reduced blood flow and reduced metabolic activity in the feet that will reduce healing capacity and promote degeneration.

If you have a job that requires exposure to cold temperatures for hours on end, then quit. If you live in a cold environment, you may want to think about moving to a warmer climate.

Thyroid Dysfunction

Thyroid hormones control metabolic activity and regulate the temperature of the body. The feet are far from the heart, so they are usually colder and less metabolically active than the rest of the body. If you have a thyroid disorder, especially hypothyroidism, your foot health will be detrimentally affected. People who have hypothyroidism will usually have weak toenails and skin on the feet.

If your thyroid hormones are off, your body temperature will fluctuate by a degree or more. Considering that the feet are already colder than other areas of the body, thyroid issues can cause many other problems in the feet. Healing capacity and ability to fight infections will be detrimentally affected. The feet will have a limited supply of nutrients, and waste products can accumulate in the feet, causing further problems.

Find a way to fix your thyroid without drugs. If you have hypothyroidism, start taking iodine and selenium every day, and reduce exposure to toxic chemicals that hurt the thyroid gland (such as chlorine, fluoride, and bromines). If you have an auto-immune thyroid disorder, fix your diet.

How to Fix Weak Feet

Step One: Diet

Fix the diet first, so that your body has the raw materials to restructure and strengthen your feet:

Avoid all forms of processed foods (organic or not) and fill your diet with:

- Raw Organic Fruits and Vegetables

- Raw Organic Oils

- Sprouted Organic Nuts and Seeds

- Organic animal products that do not emphasize the meat. Meat lacks nutrients. Bones/organs/brains/eggs/liver is extremely dense in nutrients.

- Fermented Foods

- Herbs and Spices

- Unrefined salt. Celtic sea salt is ideal

- Clean filtered water stored in glass or stainless steel

We will also need specific nutrients to promote bone building in the feet to avoid injury from strengthening the feet. We will supply these nutrients to our bodies with supplements. Keep in mind that supplements are made to "supplement" a healthy diet. If you do not have a good diet, supplements do not have much effect.

List of required supplements:

1. **Vitamin A and D from an animal source:** The best source of these two nutrients is cod liver oil. Eating liver is an excellent way to consume Vitamin A, and sun exposure is the best way to make Vitamin D.
2. **Magnesium:** Ionic magnesium is most ideal. If that is not available, then use chelated forms. Take 400mg to 600mg a day.
3. **Vitamin K2 (MK7):** Find a K2 MK7 supplement that does not contain fillers. Take 150mcg-200mcg. Cultured Organic Ghee from Pasture Raised/Grass Fed Cows and Natto are great sources of food based K2.

> 4. **Trace Mineral Concentrate:** My favorite is Concentrace© by Trace Mineral Research.
>
> 5. **Calcium:** No one should consume synthetic calcium supplements. You need to derive this nutrient from your diet. It is easy to find, and supplementation of synthetic calcium can cause problems. Dark leafy greens such as chard and kale are filled with calcium. Excellent animal sources of calcium are sardines and bone broth.

These supplements should be supplied by your diet, but in this world that we live in, our soil is depleted of nutrients, and supplementation of nutrients is required.

Many synthetic vitamins and overly processed minerals can cause further problems. Stick to the list above and if you can, try to find these nutrients in food sources.

Foods that you should always avoid:

- Processed foods of all kinds. This includes packaged foods that are not fresh, pasteurized juices, bread and pasta, most canned foods, frozen foods, microwave dinners, etc. This stuff is not real food!
- Fake Oils: Hydrogenated/Partially Hydrogenated Oils. These do not belong inside humans.
- Refined Carbohydrates: Sugar, Glucose, Dextrose, High Fructose Corn Syrup and Fruit Juices. Just because it is "organic evaporated cane juice" does not mean it is healthy. (Agave syrup may be low glycemic, but it is high in glycemic load. Avoid all sweeteners except for stevia.)
- Dairy products. Cow's milk is for baby cows. Goat's milk is for baby goats. Human consumption of dairy products is illogical. It can cause changes in your hormones, and can leech minerals from your body. Avoid at all costs.
- Corn oil/Soy oil/Canola oil/Cottonseed oil/Safflower oil
- Grains/Flours/Gluten free flours/Rice. Just because something is gluten-free does not make it healthy! Most gluten free products are heavily processed and cause health issues.
- Cooked oils. Coconut oil, ghee and palm oil should be the only oils you cook with. Most oils, especially polyunsaturated oils, are extremely unhealthy to consume after you cook them. People think they are making a healthy choice by using olive oil. Olive oil is only healthy when it is raw. If you heat it up, it becomes toxic.
- Cooked vegetables. Raw is much healthier.
- Synthetic vitamins. Bioavailability (how much you can absorb of a nutrient) is very small from synthetic vitamins. To absorb vitamins, one must eat whole foods that contain

them. Some vitamins can be absorbed if they are a "food-based formulation" that provides all of the necessary components for absorbing the vitamins.

- White table salt. It is toxic, and no one should consume it!
- Anything containing caffeine. Caffeine is bad for multiple organ systems, especially the adrenal glands and the brain. Avoiding caffeine also includes avoidance of green tea/herbal teas with caffeine/coffee and more. Do not consume it! Just because something comes from a plant does not mean it is good for you. Avoid it at all cost.
- Protein powders. If you want protein, eat a whole food that contains it.
- Factory farmed eggs/meat/fish.
- MSG and food preservatives. If you avoid processed foods entirely, you should be able to avoid these easily.
- Processed lunch meats and heavily processed sausages.
- Drugs and alcohol. They are not ideal substances to have in the human body.

You want to buy foods that have ingredients that you are familiar with. If there are any strange names or long words, then it is more than likely a synthetic additive or preservative. Lots of health foods have added things such as "natural flavors" or "natural colors." Your food should only contain real food that is found in nature. It should contain a couple ingredients that you know of. The best foods are the ones that have one ingredient.

Many people will look at the list of foods and think "wow! I cannot eat anything now!" That is far from the truth. There are millions of food choices that do not fit into the previously mentioned categories. Most grocery stores are filled with food that is not fit for human consumption. Many people were raised to think that these foods are made for humans, so making changes to most people's diet, can be as radical as changing their religion. The best way to look at it is to say "what does my body need?"

Do not try to find replacements for foods that you cannot eat. Many people, when told to avoid something, attempt to find a way around it. If they cannot eat gluten, they seek out gluten free bread (even though it is still processed and unhealthy). If someone wants to avoid meat, they will make "vegan burgers", which are nearly always unhealthy. If you cannot find a healthy alternative, do not eat it. I understand that people are used to eating bread/pasta/burgers/pizza, and will try to find healthy alternatives. You can attempt to do this, but usually, it is a lot easier to find new recipes that accommodate a nutritious diet. Raw foodist's and paleo recipe books have plenty of great ideas. I am personally lazy and hate preparing food. Instead of making a salad, I just put the vegetables in my mouth and eat them. It is way faster, and I get the nutrients my body so craves.

Step Two: Bone Alignment/Release Trigger Points
Get rid of Orthotics

Start this step on day 1 and gradually stop in 2-3 months

Before we work on strengthening the feet, we need to fix some preexisting issues. Most people have foot bones that are out of alignment and active trigger points in their muscles (Trigger points are muscle knots that are tender to massage. A trigger point is a chronic contraction of muscle that can cause pain and circulation issues in the feet and sometimes other areas of the body). If the bones and muscles are not working properly, you cannot strengthen the feet. You can exercise your feet all day long, but your results will be limited if the bones and muscles are not functioning properly. The reason that your bones and muscles are dysfunctional is due to a lifetime of wearing shoes. We want to progressively fix this problem to avoid injury.

How to align the bones of the foot:

Wear toe spreading devices such as Correct Toes©, silicone toe spreaders, and toe spreading socks. These devices will push the foot bones into a proper alignment. The secret to using them is a slow progression. Moving the bones of your feet will cause many changes in your entire body. This step should be a gradual and day by day progression. Persistence and effort will be required. Start by wearing these toe spreading devices when you are at home, or while sitting down. Begin by wearing them for an hour or so on the first day, and then slowly increase the time that you wear them. If you begin to feel pain from doing this step, give it a break and come back to it when the pain is gone.

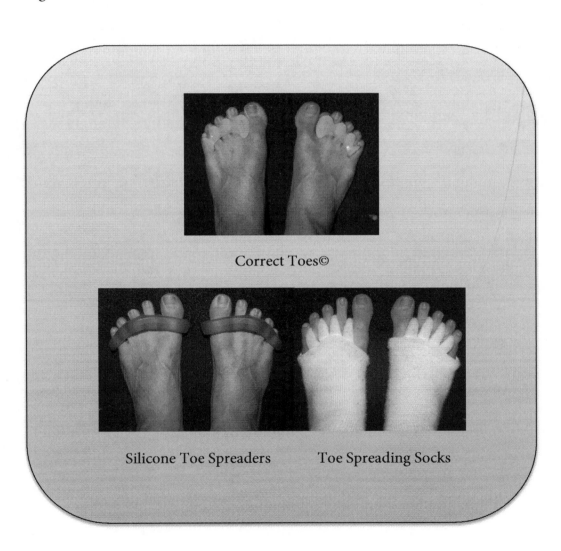

Correct Toes©

Silicone Toe Spreaders   Toe Spreading Socks

You also need to do specific stretches daily to align the bones of the feet. These stretches should be gentle. Do not try to force anything! If it hurts, you need to stop.

Stretch One: Toe Separation

Take the big toe and stretch it away from the other toes. This needs to be an extremely gentle stretch! Do not force the stretch. With time and persistence, the big toe will move away from the other toes. You do not want the joint of the big toe to stretch that much. If you have a bunion, you will need to work this stretch often. Hold for 60 seconds every day.

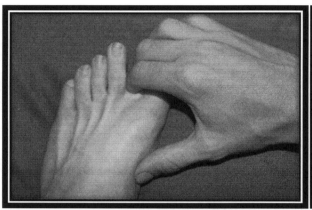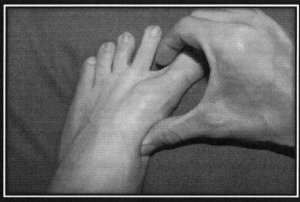

The next method will also aim at stretching the big toe, but is a bit different. You need to support the big toe from its base, next to its joint, so that you can spread the bones of the foot apart. This stretch is safer than the stretch above, and you can add more pressure. Do not force the stretch! Nice and easy. Hold for 60 seconds every day.

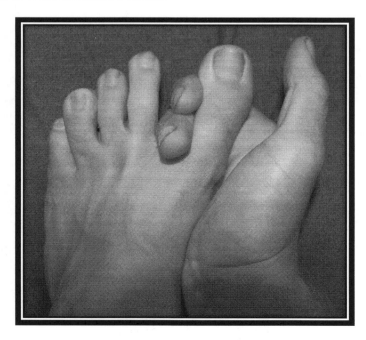

These stretches will open the spaces between the foot bones. You want all the foot bones to stretch away from each other so that the foot can return to its natural shape.

Each toe separation stretch should be held for 10 seconds.

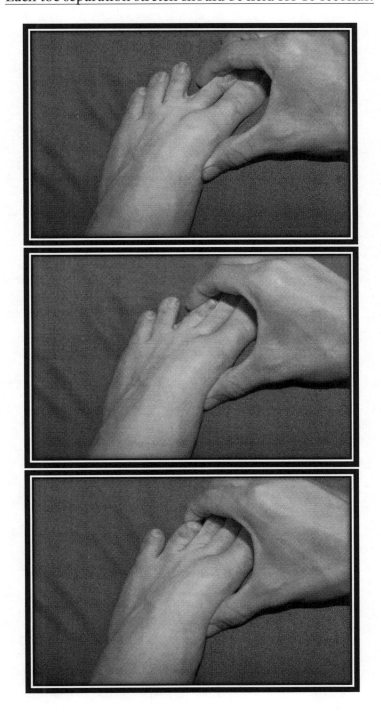

These stretches can also start at the pinky toe instead of the big toe:

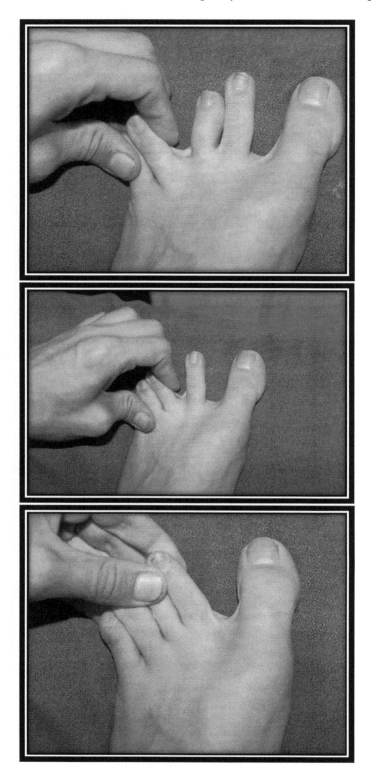

While you stand and walk, you should focus on spreading your toes. If you are doing the stretches above and wearing toe spreading devices, your toe muscles will start to adapt to the new position. You will be able to spread your toes at any time. Be sure to wear shoes that have room for you to spread your toes outward.

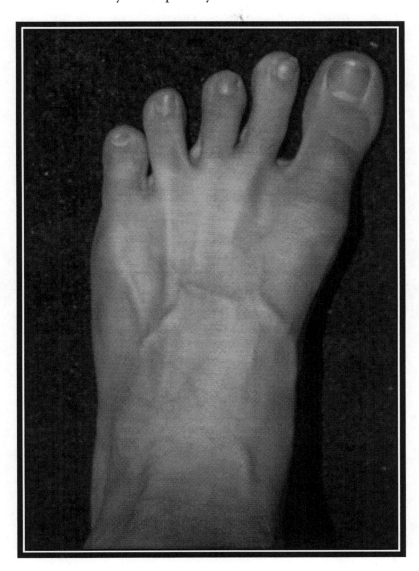

Stretch Two: Toe Flexion

Shoes bring the toes upward in the front of the shoe. This is called toe spring. Having the toes chronically lifted will cause the muscles on the bottom of your foot to be chronically stretched, and weak. These muscles are important because they support the arch of your foot. If you do not fix this problem, your foot muscles will stay weak. You need to stretch the toes downward so that the arch muscles can once again function properly.

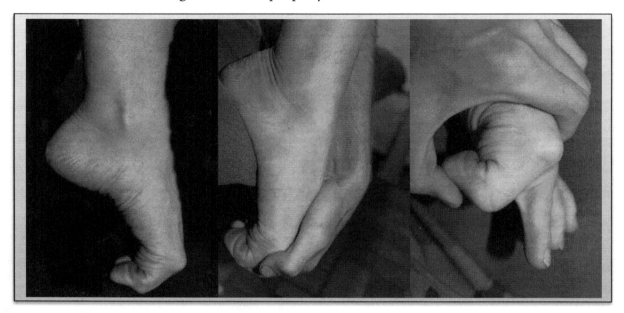

The first stretch can be done while sitting down or standing up. Put the top of your toes on the ground, and gently stretch them downward. (First Picture on Left)

The second stretch requires putting your heel on the edge of a bed or a chair. Point the toes down and use your hands to manually stretch the toes further. This is my favorite stretch toe flexion stretch. (Middle Picture)

The third stretch requires isolating the big toe and stretching it downward. (Last Picture on Right)

Pick either the first or second stretch, and hold it for 60 seconds, and then do the third stretch for 30 seconds. Repeat every day.

How to fix the Trigger Points:

A few of the muscles in your body have trigger points that you need to take care of before you work on strengthening your feet. Most of the trigger points will be found in these muscles:

- Calves
- Hamstrings
- Hip Flexors
- Back Muscles

The best way to find the trigger points is to massage the muscles and find areas that are tender and hurt to rub (muscle knots). When we find a trigger point, we want to slowly rub it with a deep and strong force. When it is less tender, or the muscle itself feels softer, then we know we are done. Many trigger points will release with a deep and forceful rub of 6 to 12 slow strokes.

Sometimes you will not only find a tender spot, but you might find a small nodule, lump or tight band in the muscle as well. This is what a trigger point feels like.

You need to slowly massage this trigger point out until it is not as tender as when you started. Rubbing them back and forth is the best way to do this. Rub them nice and slow. If you apply too much pressure to these little trigger points, you will have more pain and more problems. If you massage them nice and softly and have a medium amount of pain while doing so, you will ultimately have less pain and fewer problems. If you do not feel a tender spot, try pushing harder and deeper into the tissues. Sometimes they like to hide pretty deep inside a muscle.

Sometimes rubbing a trigger point will generate a "good pain", like when you get knots massaged out of your back. The key to releasing trigger points is to not apply too much pressure. When you massage the trigger points, do not go more than 6 out of 10 on the pain scale, where 0 is no pain, and 10 is the most pain.

Do not overdo it! It is much better to keep at 6 out of 10 on the pain scale and do a lot of consistent small sessions of trigger point work than it is to do an inconsistent number of "hard" sessions. 3 small sessions a day is much better for you than 1 hard session once a day.

Using tools will allow you to use more pressure on a trigger point than you can with just your hands. I also suggest trying to use tools whenever you can to avoid using your thumbs. Thumbs can be damaged by using them to rub out trigger points.

After a few sessions of trigger point therapy, you may feel like your tender spots have become less sensitive and that you might be fine without any more trigger point work. This is wrong. Keep feeling the muscles and search for new trigger points. Sometimes after doing the superficial (surface) layer of muscles, you will later find a whole new set of trigger points deeper in the muscle. These will usually require more focused pressure to release them. If you do not see results, try pushing a bit harder. Just keep with it daily and do not give up!

You can do these trigger point release methods any time throughout the day. If the area becomes extremely sore or feels more tender, let the area rest and come back to it in a day or two. Your body will adapt to the trigger point therapy quickly, and it is not unusual for you to be able to double the number of therapy sessions and pressure that you use on the trigger points in as little as 2-3 weeks. It is important to ease slowly into the treatments and to build up to more sessions and more pressure while massaging. Listen to your body and respond accordingly.

How to release the Calf Muscles

The trigger points in this muscle group will be the most important to release if you want strong feet. Due to shoes causing the heel to be elevated, many people have shortened calf muscles for years. It can take months to release the trigger points in the calf muscle. As your feet become stronger over time, check the calves to see if they develop further trigger points.

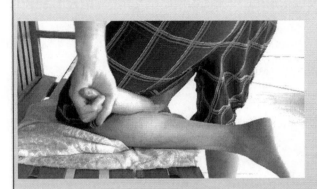

Put your lower leg and knee on the side of a bed or soft surface and use a rolling pin to roll out the trigger points in this muscle group.

Use a foam roller to release the calf muscle trigger points. Push the calf muscle directly into the foam roller, and then point and flex your foot. Do slow, strong passes over the entire muscle group.

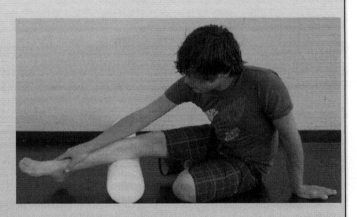

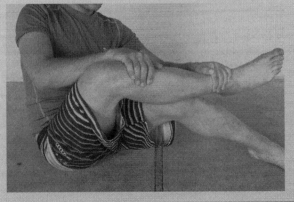

Put one calf muscle over the opposite legs knee and let the weight of your leg dig into the other legs calf muscle. This can get rid of deep trigger points in the calves. The picture shows me doing this method while sitting on the floor, but it is easier for most people to do it will sitting in a chair.

How to release the Hamstrings

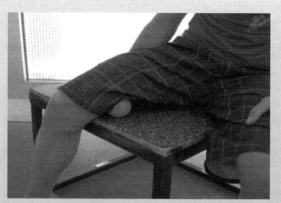

Use two lacrosse balls on a flat bench to roll out any trigger points you find. This is a big muscle and finding the trigger points requires some patience. Watch out for the Sciatic nerve near the upper portion of the muscle (near the butt). It is very sensitive and painful if you hit the Sciatic nerve with a lacrosse ball. Try to stay in the belly of the muscle.

You can also use a small foam roller to roll out these muscles if they are too sensitive to be worked out with the lacrosse balls.

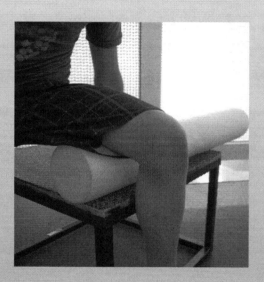

How to release the Hip Flexors

If you are skinny or healthy without too much abdominal fat, this muscle can be treated with your hands.

This muscle is under your organs and on the back wall of your stomach cavity. If you cannot reach the muscle because you are overweight, then skip this muscle. There is a hip flexor stretch that is coming up that you will need to work on instead.

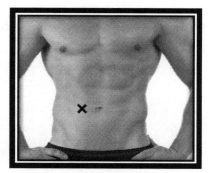

Location of Muscle

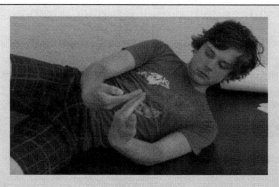

Put your hands into what is known as the Supported Finger Technique

Lay on the ground, on your back with your knees bent at 90 degree angles and your feet flat on the ground. Put one hand's finger's 1 inch to either side of your belly button and push your fingers into your stomach slowly. Feel around for a hot-dog shaped muscle, and press into it. Once you push into the muscle, it may be tender. This is a trigger point. Try to rub it out…

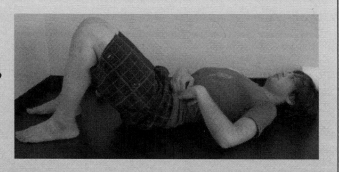

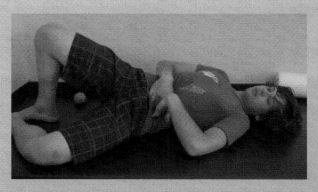

While rubbing the muscle, try to relax the leg on the side being treated and let it slowly fall to the ground. Then while still applying pressure to the muscle, bring the leg up to the beginning position, and then repeat.

Repeat on the other side of the body.

How to release the Back Muscles

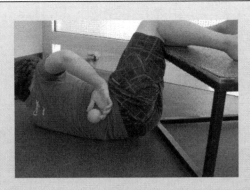

Use one or two lacrosse balls to release the back muscle's trigger points. Put them on the ground and roll your back over them slowly (picture shows the placement of lacrosse ball).

It is even better to put your feet up on a small box (as pictured) or chair so that the muscles relax even further. Do not use a foam roller on the lower back.

Another great way to get the trigger points to release is with The Back Buddy© stick. This stick gets right in the areas you want, and you can use the stick as a lever to push a lot of mechanical pressure into the area.

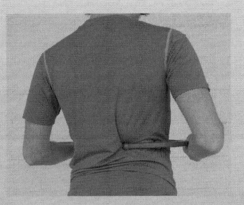

Another tool that I love to release the back muscles with is an electric shiatsu massage chair. These tools, unlike our hands, never get tired. For an added effect, lay the massage chair on the ground so that you have to put your whole weight on the chair, and then let the massage chair work out any trigger points it finds.

Once you release the trigger points in these muscle groups, they will function properly, and this will cause the bones to re-align into their natural and functional position. When the bones are aligned, and the trigger points are taken care of, the muscles will instantly be stronger, and your feet and legs will have improved healing abilities. It will also improve circulation and nerve function.

There is one final step to releasing the trigger points. After treating the trigger points for about 2 weeks, you will also want to stretch the muscles, so that the results of the trigger point therapy can stay.

The stretches that we are about to do are not common stretches. They are aimed at stretching multiple groups of muscles, or "kinetic chains". This will require you to stretch multiple joints simultaneously.

Many stretches that are practiced today cause damage because they put your joints into unstable positions. Forcing a joint into an unnatural and unstable position will cause many joint issues. The stretches about to be mentioned will prevent this problem because they focus on stretching a specific kinetic chain. This puts tension only where it is needed without stressing the joints. When the entire kinetic chain is stretched, the joints can only move in their natural range of motion and no further.

These stretches are listed on the following pages and should be done daily, after the trigger point therapy.

Calf Stretch

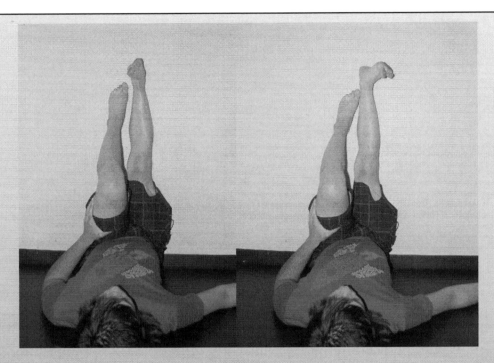

- Lie down next to a wall and kick your feet up against the wall.

- Push your butt into the wall slowly.

- Flatten your back by contracting your abs.

- Extend the knee joint on the side being stretched. This is done by contracting the quadriceps.

- Bring the toes and foot back towards your face.

- While doing this stretch, there are two variations. One is inverted, the other is everted. Inverted means that the bottom of the foot is facing towards the opposite leg. Everted means that the bottom of the foot is facing away from the opposite leg.

- Invert the foot while doing this stretch for 20 seconds (picture on the left shows how to invert the foot). Then evert the foot while doing this stretch for 20 seconds (picture on right shows how to evert the foot). Rest for 20 seconds. Then choose whichever stretch was harder (inverted or everted) and stretch that position for another 20 seconds.

Hamstring Stretches

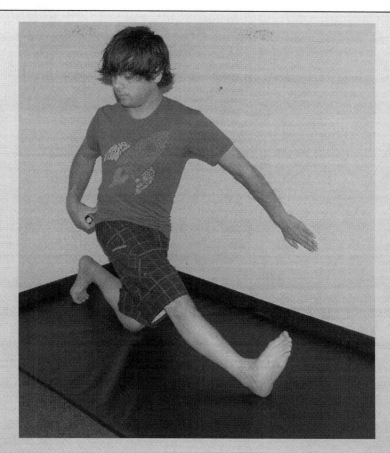

Outer Hamstring Stretch:

- Assume position in the picture.

- Invert foot (point the bottom of the foot towards the opposite leg).

- Extend the foot up towards the sky while inverting it. Do not try to stretch the calf; you should feel only a small stretch in the calf while doing this.

- Next, contract the quadriceps muscles to straighten and extend the knee joint.

- Lift up your chest and then slowly lower your stomach and torso down to the leg being stretched. Also, slowly rotate the chest towards the leg being stretched. Slowly bring your chest further down to the leg while contracting the quadriceps so that the hamstring muscles will release.

- Hold this stretch for 20 seconds, then rest for 10 seconds, then stretch again for 30 seconds.

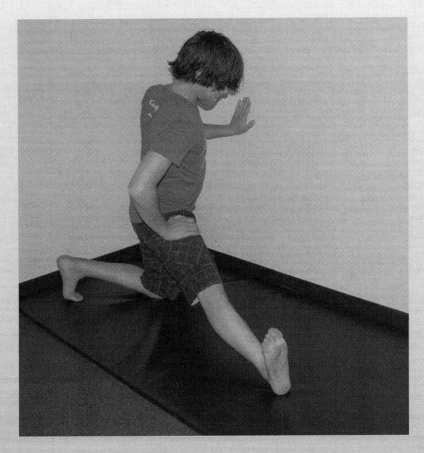

Inner Hamstring Stretch:

- Assume position in the picture.

- Evert foot (point the bottom of the foot away from the midline of the body; outward).

- Extend the foot up towards the sky while everting it. Do not try to stretch the calf; you should feel only a small stretch in the calf while doing this.

- Next, contract the quadriceps muscles to straighten and extend the knee joint.

- Lift up your chest and then slowly lower your stomach and torso down to the leg being stretched. Also, slowly rotate the chest away from the leg being stretched.

- Slowly bring your stomach further down to the leg while contracting the quadriceps so that the hamstring muscles will release.

- Hold this stretch for 20 seconds, then rest for 10 seconds, then stretch again for 30 seconds.

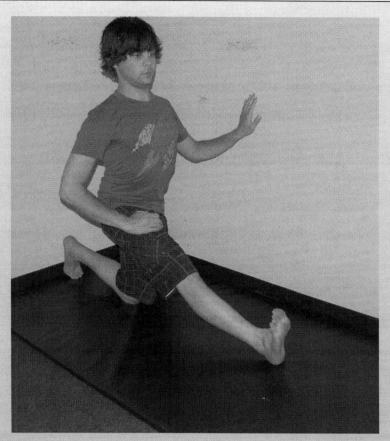

Middle Hamstring Stretch:

- Assume position in the picture.

- Extend the foot up towards the sky. Do not try to stretch the calf; you should feel only a small stretch in the calf while doing this.

- Next, contract the quadriceps muscles to straighten and extend the knee joint.

- Lift up your chest and then slowly lower your stomach and torso down to the leg being stretched.

- Slowly bring your chest further down to the leg while contracting the quadriceps so that the hamstring muscles will release.

- Hold this stretch for 20 seconds, then rest for 10 seconds, then stretch again for 30 seconds.

Hip Flexor Stretch

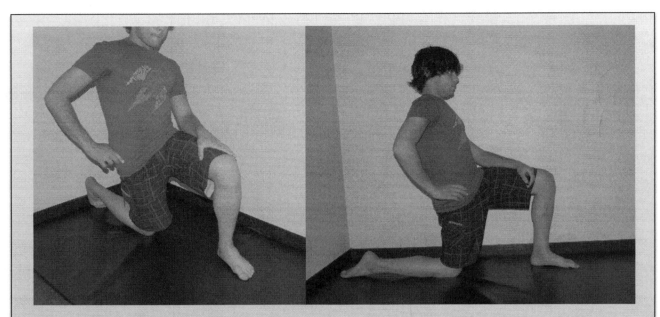

- Assume the position in the picture above.

- Make sure that you have a piece of soft padding or foam under your knee. Pillows work for this purpose.

- Make a slight double chin and keep your chest up and back straight.

- Now the important part: Contract the abdominals and glutes so that the hip flexors will release and stretch.

- Tilt your upper body away from the side being stretched (away from the leg that is behind you).

- The back foot may drift towards the opposite side of the body. You need to keep it straight behind you. You can prevent this by using a wall or stationary object to put against the inner edge of the foot that is behind you.

- Hold the stretch for 20 seconds, relax for 10, and then hold for another 30 seconds.

Back Stretch

This stretch will release the muscles and ligaments in the lower back. Do not do this stretch if your lower back pain is severe or if you have active sciatica!

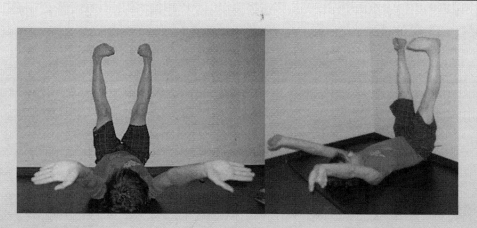

- Assume the position in the picture above. Lie down on the floor next to a wall, and then swing your legs up against the wall.

- Lift head slightly off the ground, make a double chin, but do not bend your neck. You want your spine to be straight, and this is only done by making a double chin without bending your neck. Moreover, when you lift your head off the ground, it should be less than an inch, not much.

- Push your legs down into your pelvis. You need to imagine your legs sinking into your pelvis. Let gravity push them slowly into position while you are against the wall.

- Invert the feet (point the bottom of the feet towards your midline).

- Lock the knees by contracting the Quadriceps muscles. Also, while inverting your feet, try to bring them towards your knee (extend them).

- Internally rotate your legs. Do this by trying to point your knees forward or towards each other. Or by pointing your feet at each other (this should be a subtle rotation, not very extreme, look at the pictures and notice how my feet are pointing at each other slightly).

- Tighten your abdominals so that your back is flat on the ground.

- Push your arms above your head with your fingers extended and your elbows locked and straight.

- Hold for 30 seconds, relax for 10, and then hold for 30 more seconds. Do not forget to breathe! Do not hold your breath while doing this stretch.

Get rid of Orthotics or Arch Support:

If you are wearing any form of arch support, such as an orthotic, this is the time to slowly get rid of it. Progressively wear your orthotic for fewer hours every day. For example, on the first day, take your orthotic or arch support out of your shoe for about an hour, and then the next day, 2 hours. If you start to feel pain, take a break and wear the orthotic for a few days. If you do not have any pain from taking out the orthotic, then gradually get rid of it. Even if you have no pain at all, make this change a slow and progressive change.

Step Three: Strengthen the Foot Muscles

Avoid Sitting Down/ Wear Less Supportive Shoes

Start this step at 2-3 months and continue the methods until you can walk all day without sore feet

After you have fixed your diet, aligned the bones of the feet, released the trigger points and removed the orthotics/arch support from your shoes, you are now ready for the next step! You may continue the trigger point treatments if they still help, but you want to stop doing them eventually. If your trigger points are still around after 2-3 months, you could have a hormone disorder or your diet is to blame.

In step 3, we will start to see some awesome results. Now that we have the bones in position, and the muscles are firing properly, we can now strengthen the structures of the feet. In the next few months, you will be "reconnected" with your feet. You will be able to use them in ways that you never thought possible before. Your feet will not be sore from walking all day, and they will heal faster and feel stronger. You may notice that your posture will improve, and your feet will feel quick and agile. Some people may find that their preexisting knee/back/neck pain has suddenly disappeared or has greatly improved.

How to strengthen the foot muscles

The first exercise can be done while standing with your shoes off. Simply press your big toe into the ground, and lift up the toes as high as you can. This will be hard to do at first. With a few minutes of practice, you should be able to do it. Focus on pushing the big toe downward, and also outward, away from the other toes. Try to lift the small toes as high as you can. Do this exercise until you feel a good burn, and then stop. Repeat until the muscles are fatigued.

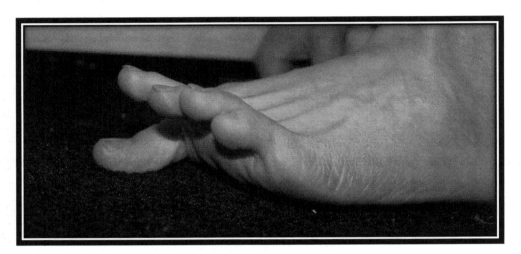

In this exercise, we will press the toes into the ground, and lift the big toe. Try to extend your big toe as high as you can. This will cause some cramping in the muscles. Do this exercise until you feel some cramping and fatigue, and then stop. Repeat until foot muscles are tired.

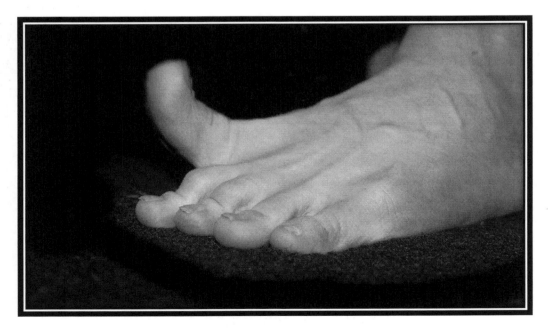

The next exercise will require a bit more effort than the previous ones. While standing barefoot, press all of your toes into the ground. Tilt your body forward and push yourself back with only your toes. You also want to focus on spreading the toes when you do this exercise. Repeat this exercise until you feel a good burn, and then stop. This picture shows my toes pushing into the ground:

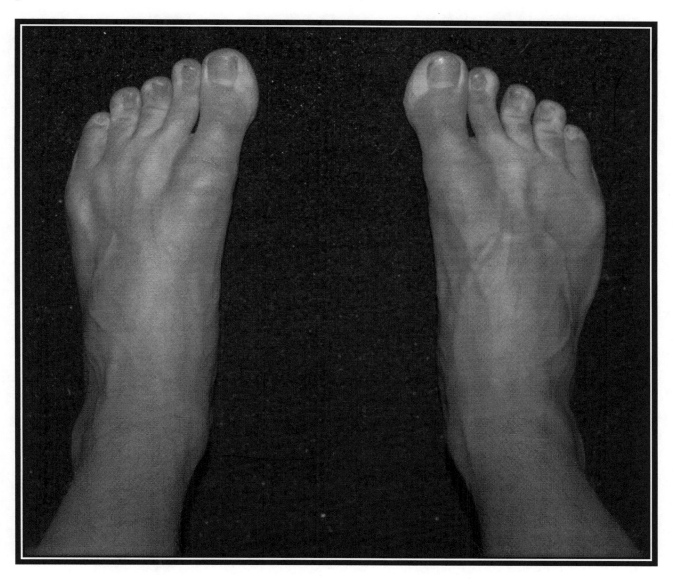

Now we will focus on strengthening the lower leg muscles. You will do calf raises with your feet pointing inward and outward. Repeat this exercise until you feel a good burn, and then stop. Repeat until the muscles are fatigued:

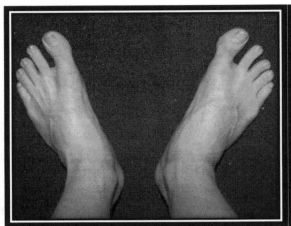 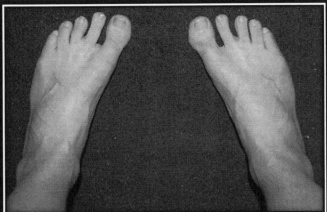

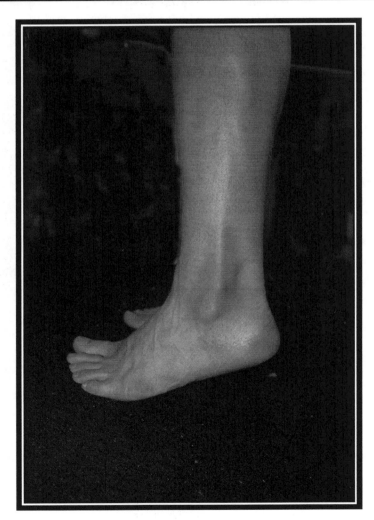

Now we want to work out the muscles in the shin (the ankle extensors). Find a wall and lean your back against it while standing. Position your feet so that your heels are 12 inches away from the wall. Now lift up your foot as shown in the picture below. Repeat this exercise until you feel a burn in your shin muscles.

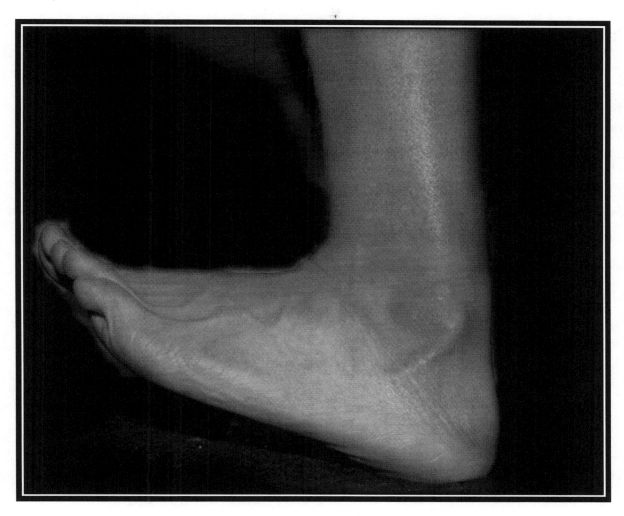

How to avoid sitting down

You need to adjust your living habitat and workplace to enable standing. You cannot sit down all day long and not expect problems to develop. If you have a desk job, buy a standing desk. These will work with your pre-existing desk and will allow you to work on your computer without a chair.

Try to avoid driving as much as possible. If you have to drive or sit on a plane or train often, then get up and move every 20 minutes or so. Sitting down for more than 30 minutes at a time is asking for problems. If you can, get up and move around every couple of minutes. Do not stop moving!

You need to start this step after you have prepared your feet and started exercising them. If your feet are not prepared, and you suddenly start to stand all day long, your feet are going to hurt. Standing all day will cause your feet to be sore at first, but if it is painful, you are progressing too quickly. Give it a break and slow down. Work on the foot exercises and stretches, and increase your standing time gradually, day by day.

How to transition to less supportive shoes

So you understand that shoes are bad, but you obviously need to wear shoes. You do not want to step on glass or a nail, so you need to find shoes that allow your feet to function properly, and still offer protection. You also do not want to wear shoes that look too crazy (some minimal shoes look somewhat strange). Many people have jobs that require them to follow dress codes. Luckily there are shoes that look completely normal and promote healthy feet!

The best place to purchase less supportive shoes is the internet. Search for "Minimal Shoes" to see what options you have. My favorite minimal shoe companies are:

- Lems© (The best all-around minimal shoe that looks completely normal!)
- Vivo Barefoot©
- Altra©
- Vibram Five Fingers©
- ZEMGear©

All of these shoes have features that let your feet function in their natural position. If you want to find a minimal shoe at a local shoe store, be sure that the shoe has these features:

- Flexible sole. You should be able to roll the shoe up, or bend it at any section of the sole.
- No heel elevation. The shoe should allow your foot to be entirely flat, with your heel planted on the ground.
- No Arch Support
- Wide Toe Box
- Loose all around. Do not wear a shoe that requires you to tie your shoe laces very tight. You want your foot to have room to expand and contract with every step.
- No toe spring. If the shoe lifts your toes up in the front of the shoe, pass on it. You need the foot to be completely flat.

After you find a minimal shoe to wear, you want to make a slow transition to wearing it. Wear the shoes on and off for about a month, progressively using them more and more. Do not take off your current shoes and throw them away. Adjusting to minimal shoes can take some time if you do not want to be injured. Start with one hour of wearing minimal shoes the first day, and then 1.5 hours the next day. Slowly over a few months, your feet will adapt to the shoes and then you can wear them all day long without any problems.

At first, wear them at home or work, and avoid using them while working out. Do not put your minimal shoes on and go for a run. Your feet are not strong enough for this quite yet. Give it a few months of time and you will be able to run pain-free with your minimal shoes.

If you start to develop pain under your big toe joint, or the top of the foot, you will need a metatarsal pad. These are inexpensive pads that you can find at most stores or the internet.

Step Four: Maintaining Foot Strength

Begin this step at 5-6 months. If you are healthy and progressed through the previous steps quickly, then you can start this step when it feels right to you.

Once you have strengthened your feet, you are good to go! Maintaining the health and strength of your feet is very easy because all you need to do is walk often. Walking feels much nicer when your feet are strong, so you will now be able to walk as much as you like. Daily walks that last for more than an hour are a great way to stay active and avoid development of common health problems. These walks are also a convenient time to increase your sun exposure.

If you want to make your feet extremely strong, walk in sand or on uneven surfaces. Find tall grass that requires you to lift your feet up high. Walk up and down big hills.

When can I run?
Many people's bodies and feet are not strong enough to run. After you have developed the ability to stand on your feet all day long without pain, you are now ready to run. Running on natural surfaces is more ideal, but only when the feet are strong. If you have weak feet and run on grass, you will develop problems. Running on natural surfaces require muscle and bone strength that develops over time.

Advanced Foot Strength Exercises

So far this book has dealt with fixing foot problems and regaining strength required for daily activities. If you are an athlete or simply care about your health, follow the exercises on the following pages to make your feet extremely strong.

One Leg Balance

This is a simple exercise, but doing it with correct form requires some practice. You will want to contract your abdominal muscles and glutes, and push your toes into the ground. Notice how my toes are spread outward, and my arch is raised in the photos below. If you do not have proper form while doing this exercise, you can develop problems. You can do this exercise while standing in line at the store, waiting for people and while brushing your teeth. If you want to make this exercise extremely difficult, close your eyes while doing it. If you are older or have vestibular dysfunction or random bouts of vertigo, you should be very careful. Try to hold this position for as long as possible. If the arch of the foot collapses, or your pelvis starts to tilt forward, then you should stop. This exercise becomes easier after about a week of doing it every day.

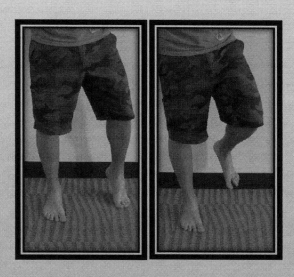

One Leg Calf Raises

This exercise is more advanced than balancing on one foot. You should practice standing on one foot with your eyes closed for a few weeks before attempting this exercise.

A strong posture is required while doing this exercise, which means having the arch of the foot raised and the toes splayed out, and your pelvis in a good position.

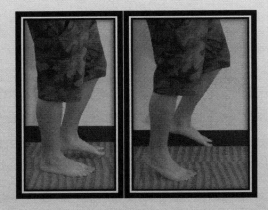

Do this exercise until the muscles are fatigued, and then stop. Be mindful of the arch of your foot and the tilt of your pelvis. If your posture starts to weaken while doing this exercise, you need to stop. You are not strong enough to do more.

You can do this exercise at random times throughout the day. If you have balance problems, hold onto a wall or a chair.

Full Range Body Squat

This is a basic and foundational exercise that all humans should practice daily. In many cultures around the world, people relax and sit in a full squat. Many of these people do not use chairs. This position aligns many structures of the body. It puts a natural amount of stretch to specific muscles, and it puts joints into healthy positions.

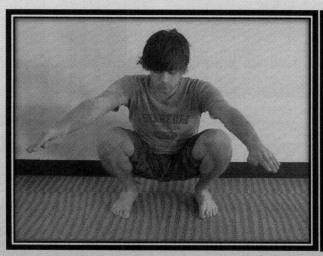 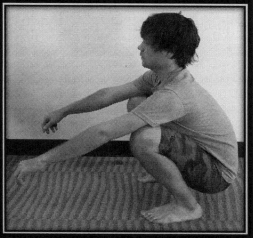

Take notice of my posture. My big toes are pointed somewhat inward, and my arch is raised because I am contracting the small muscles on the bottom of my foot by pressing my toes into the ground. This will force the lower leg bones to be in a proper position for a healthy squat. If your arches collapse and your knees go inward, then you need to take a step back and focus on strengthening the foot muscles and sorting out any muscular imbalances as mentioned before.

If you are not athletic, and your body cannot safely do a basic squat, then you should start by doing squats while holding onto a metal pole or other sturdy object. In the picture below, I am holding onto a door handle and doing a squat. This will put less stress on your joints, and you will not have to stretch your muscles as much to achieve a squat.

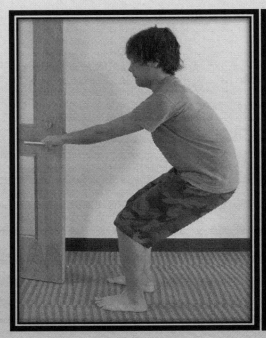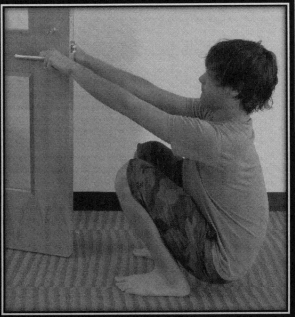

Try to squat at random times of the day. If you find yourself in a situation where you need to kill time, squat down and relax in this position. Many people will find that their muscles are short and this causes their heel to be slightly raised. Make it your goal to be able to do this movement with your heel planted on the ground. Go back to the stretches mentioned previously to fix this problem. Use the previously mentioned "Calf Stretch" to make the full body squat possible.

Morton's Toe

Morton's toe is a common developmental fault that is seen in 10% of the population. This means that the toe next to your big toe is longer than the big toe (take your shoes off and take a look). This can impose a few detrimental issues to walking gait mechanics. It is easily fixed with a pad under the big toe (which can be found at pharmacy stores and the internet).

Some doctors will tell you that it is a huge issue, and some doctors will say that it does not matter much. It is somewhat confusing to draw a solid conclusion on the significance of this problem when everyone is saying something different. Some cases are obviously more severe than others. If you have localized pain or callous formation under your 2nd toe (the long toe), then you may need to see a holistic podiatrist. Most people do not need to do that and report benefits from a simple Morton's toe pad that is available at the store.

I think that the bigger issue that we need to look at is how Morton's toe develops. It is seen as a congenital disorder, which means that it was created before birth. Is it due to faulty genes or expression of unfavorable genes? It is hard to say, but there is a commonality among people with Morton's toe:

They seem to have a problem converting vitamin B6 to its active and usable form. What this means is that a person with Morton's toe can develop a vitamin B6 deficiency, regardless of how much B6 they consume in their diet. This can cause skin/hair/nail and nerve problems. B6 is required for many processes in the body, and the body can be detrimentally affected by a B6 deficiency.

Usually, when people come to me complaining of hair loss, skin and nail problems, and depression/anxiety, I look at their feet. If they have Morton's toe, then I know that their B6 conversion process is not working properly.

Luckily we live in a time that we can solve this problem with supplementation. Humans have isolated the active form of B6, which is P5P. So if you have Morton's toe and nail/hair/skin/nerve/brain issues, find a P5P supplement at the store.

I am sure that there is more to this problem than we know at the present time, but it is hard to say with current technology. Hopefully we will find a solid answer to this problem soon.

Conclusion

What I wish to accomplish with my books:

- Fix people's unnecessary suffering
- Improve the physical and mental function of my readers which can have beneficial effects on society
- Improve quality of life for the children of my readers (Healthy parents usually have healthy and happy children.)

What we need to do is spread this information to people who need it. If this book helps you in any way, recommend it to your friends and family members.

If you have any questions, please email me at any time: pfsurvivalguide@gmail.com

If you have a minute to spare from your day, I would really appreciate an honest review on amazon.com for this book. I love when people tell me that they are free from pain and living a healthy life! ☺ It can also help other people find this book. Thank you!

Confused on which supplements to buy?
Check out my website to see my favorites!
Go Online and type this address into your web browser:

http://www.mstrtherapy.com/optimal-health-supplements.html

If you need relief from chronic injuries, check out:

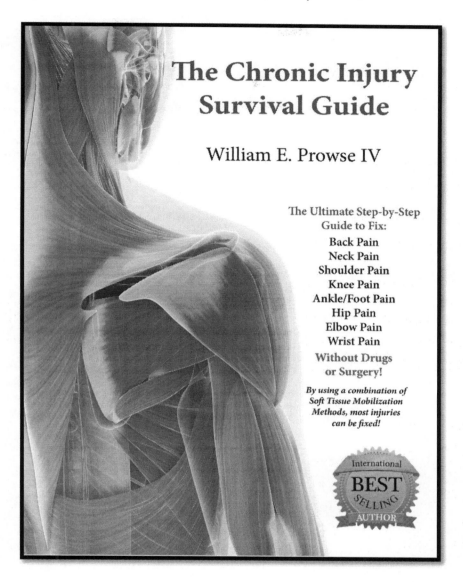

The Chronic Injury
Survival Guide

William E. Prowse IV

The Ultimate Step-by-Step
Guide to Fix:
Back Pain
Neck Pain
Shoulder Pain
Knee Pain
Ankle/Foot Pain
Hip Pain
Elbow Pain
Wrist Pain
Without Drugs
or Surgery!

*By using a combination of
Soft Tissue Mobilization
Methods, most injuries
can be fixed!*

International
BEST
SELLING
AUTHOR

Available at Amazon.com!

Fix your pain, or your money back ☺

Made in the USA
San Bernardino, CA
12 November 2016